FIFTY & THRIVING

FIFTY & THRIVING

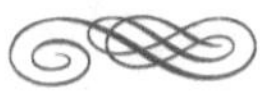

The Ultimate Nutrition Guide

B. VINCENT

QuillQuest Publishers

Contents

Introduction

As we pass the limit into our fifties, an enormous number of us begin to see changes that go past the shallow signs of developing. Our energy levels likely will not be what they used to be, recovery from dynamic work takes fairly longer, and perhaps our stomach related structures have become more sensitive. It's the place where we start to think about even more genuinely the somewhat long impact of our lifestyle choices, particularly our eating routine, on our prosperity and success.

The meaning of sustenance can't be overemphasized at any period of life, yet as we age, it transforms into a critical part in choosing the idea of our life and our opportunity. This book, "Fifty and Prospering: A conclusive Sustenance Guide," is expected to be your mate and guide through understanding and executing healthy practices that will help you with living your fifties and past effectively, yet vivaciously.

The Meaning of Sustenance as We Age

Sustenance expects a critical part in developing perfect. It's tied in with something past weight the board. Fitting food can help hinder or manage various typical diligent conditions that will regularly impact people as they age, similar to coronary ailment, diabetes, and bone thickness disaster. Past disease contravention, an especially considered diet can overhaul mental clarity, further foster energy levels, and lift immune capacity. For the most part, what you eat can through and through influence how you age.

In any case, healthy necessities change as we age. Our assimilation tones down, requiring changes in calorie affirmation. The maintenance of explicit enhancements ends up being less useful, anticipating that we should zero in on these in our eating standard or through supplementation. Additionally, our bodies could start to encourage responsive characteristics or bigotries to food assortments that we could without a doubt cycle in our more energetic years. Seeing and acclimating to these movements is crucial for staying aware of prosperity and hugeness.

Guiding You to Prosper

This book isn't just about what to eat and what to avoid. It's connected to sorting out the why behind dietary ideas and sorting out some way to make educated choices that fit your direction regarding life, tendencies, and fortifying necessities. "Fifty and Thriving" is coordinated to outfit you with comprehensive data, from the basics of food to unequivocal dietary models that advance life expectancy and vitality.

We'll research how to examine and unravel food names, the meaning of changing different nourishment classes, and when upgrades might be fundamental. We'll jump into dietary models that have been shown to help strong developing, for instance, the Mediterranean eating routine and plant-based eating, giving practical direction on the most capable technique to combine these into your everyday daily schedule. Phenomenal considerations, for instance, managing food responsive qualities and bigotries, and procedures for eating perfect regardless, when you're in a hurry, will similarly be covered.

Empowering Your Outing

We need to draw in you with the data and instruments you truly need to investigate your dietary prerequisites absolutely. Whether you're expecting to re-try your eating routine absolutely or simply go with extra instructed choices, this book will offer significant pieces of information and commonsense tips. We'll give supper orchestrating appeal, test feast plans, and recipes that take unique consideration of feeding prerequisites as well regarding the taste buds.

Developing is an undeniable piece of life, yet the way that we age is something we can affect. By making splendid healthy choices, we can ensure that our fifties and the years past are about perseverance as well as about thriving. "Fifty and Prospering: A conclusive Food Guide" is more than a book; it's a manual for a superior, more unique you.

As you leave on this outing through the pages of "Fifty and Prospering," recall that the goal isn't just to add seemingly forever to your life anyway life to your years. Sustenance is an astonishing resource in achieving that goal, and starting making changes is seldom too far to turn back. With each segment, you'll secure encounters and frameworks that will help you with investigating the many-sided universe of sustenance, tailor it to your original necessities, and embrace a superior lifestyle that maintains your best life after fifty.

I

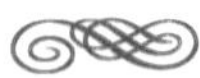

Chapter 1: The Changing Body: How Aging Affects Metabolism, Dietary Needs, and Health

As we enter our fifties, our bodies go through huge changes that can affect each part of our wellbeing and way of life, including our nourishing requirements. These progressions are a characteristic piece of maturing, yet with the right information and systems, we can relieve their belongings, guaranteeing we stay solid, dynamic, and energetic well into later life. This part dives into the points of interest of how maturing influences digestion, dietary necessities, and generally wellbeing, giving you the bits of knowledge expected to change and flourish.

The Effect of Maturing on Digestion

Digestion is the cycle by which your body changes over what you eat and drink into energy. As we age, our digestion normally dials back, a change that starts as soon as our thirties. When we arrive at our fifties, this lull can be critical, influencing how rapidly we consume calories. This diminishing in metabolic rate is part of the way because of a misfortune in bulk, which consumes a larger number of calories very still than fat does. The outcome is a propensity to put on weight all the more effectively, regardless of whether our dietary patterns haven't changed.

Understanding this shift is critical in changing our dietary admission and exercise propensities to keep a sound weight and backing generally wellbeing. It's tied in with eating less as well as about picking food varieties that are supplement thick and valuable for keeping up with bulk, like proteins and food sources plentiful in fundamental nutrients and minerals.

Dietary Necessities and Supplement Assimilation

As we age, besides the fact that our digestion eases back, however our body's capacity to retain specific supplements diminishes. This can prompt lacks in key nutrients and minerals, notwithstanding devouring similar food varieties as in the past. For example, vitamin B12, crucial for nerve capability and platelet development, becomes more diligently to assimilate. Also, calcium and vitamin D, critical for bone wellbeing, require more consideration because of diminished ingestion and the body's evolving needs.

Changing our eating routine to expand the admission of these and other fundamental supplements is important to battle these normal decays. This could mean consolidating more braced food sources, taking into account supplements under the direction of a medical care supplier, and zeroing in on various supplement rich food sources to guarantee a balanced eating regimen.

Wellbeing Contemplations

The progressions in digestion and supplement retention are joined by an expanded gamble of a few medical issue. Coronary illness, osteoporosis, and type 2 diabetes are more predominant as we age, somewhat because of changes in body structure, hormonal movements, and way of life factors. Nonetheless, sustenance can assume a strong part in forestalling and dealing with these circumstances.

For heart wellbeing, an eating routine low in soaked fats and high in fiber-rich organic products, vegetables, and entire grains is vital. To help bone wellbeing, guaranteeing sufficient admission of calcium and vitamin D, alongside taking part in weight-bearing activity, can have a tremendous effect. What's more, for glucose the executives, zeroing in on a fair eating regimen that cutoff points refined sugars and underscores entire food sources can help forestall or control diabetes.

Transformation and System

Adjusting to the body's changing necessities requires a proactive way to deal with sustenance. This includes what we eat as well as how we eat. More modest, more regular feasts can assist with overseeing digestion and energy levels all the more really. Integrating strength preparing into our activity routine can battle muscle misfortune, in a roundabout way supporting a better digestion.

It's likewise critical to pay attention to our bodies and perceive signs that healthful changes are required. Changes in energy levels, surprising weight gain or misfortune, and modifications in stomach related wellbeing can all flag that now is the ideal time to rethink our dietary propensities.

Understanding the progressions our bodies go through as we age is the most important move toward adjusting our nourishment to fulfill these new needs. By recognizing and tending to the effect of maturing on digestion, dietary requirements, and wellbeing, we can go with informed decisions that help imperativeness and health into our fifties and then some. The ensuing parts will expand on this establishment, offering nitty gritty direction on the supplements fundamental for flourishing after fifty, how to oversee normal well-being worries through diet, and useful ways to execute these techniques in day to day existence.

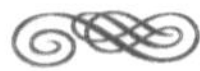

Chapter 2: Nutritional Needs After 50: Key Nutrients, Vitamins, and Minerals Essential for the Fifty-Plus Demographic

As we age, our bodies' healthy requirements create. The post-fifty years accomplish unique prosperity challenges and changes in physiological necessities, making explicit enhancements more essential than any time in late memory. This part dives into the essential supplements, minerals, and various enhancements vital to help ideal prosperity for those a bigger number of than fifty, giving significant guidance on the most capable technique to coordinate these into your eating routine.

Protein: Building and Staying aware of Mass

Mass typically declines with age, a condition known as sarcopenia, inciting lessened strength and compactness. Protein is critical for building and fixing muscle tissue, making adequate protein affirmation major for those more than fifty. Uniting an arrangement of protein sources, including lean meats, fish, poultry, vegetables, and dairy things, can help with staying aware of mass and moving in everyday actual cycles.

Calcium and Vitamin D: Supporting Bone Prosperity

Bone thickness decreases with age, growing the bet of osteoporosis and breaks. Calcium and vitamin D are integral for staying aware of bone prosperity. While calcium maintains the bones' development, vitamin D redesigns calcium maintenance and bone turn of events. Dairy things, verdant green vegetables, supported food assortments, and light receptiveness can help with meeting these enhancement necessities. In any case, improvements may be crucial for specific individuals, as recommended by a clinical benefits provider.

Fiber: Stomach related Prosperity to say the least

Fiber expects a basic part in staying aware of stomach related prosperity, which can end up being more fragile with age. It similarly adds to heart prosperity by helping with cutting down cholesterol levels and helps in supervising glucose levels. Whole grains, natural items, vegetables, and vegetables are inconceivable fiber sources, propelling a sound stomach related system and supporting all things considered prosperity.

Omega-3 Unsaturated fats: Heart Prosperity and Mental Capacity

Omega-3 unsaturated fats are central for staying aware of heart prosperity and may expect a section in saving mental capacity. Found in oily fish like salmon, mackerel, and sardines, as well as flaxseeds and walnuts, omega-3s can help with decreasing disturbance, cut down the bet of coronary disease, and sponsorship mind prosperity.

Cell fortifications: Combatting Oxidative Strain

Cell fortifications, including supplements A, C, and E, and the mineral selenium, help with combatting oxidative strain and may diminish the bet of persevering sicknesses. They similarly expect a section in supporting safe capacity and skin prosperity. An eating routine well off in natural items, vegetables, nuts, and seeds can give a vivacious load of these basic enhancements.

B Supplements: Energy, Psyche Capacity, to say the least

The B supplements, particularly B12, B6, and folate, are principal for energy creation, mind capacity, and the improvement of red platelets. Vitamin B12 ingestion decreases with age, making supplementation or the usage of reinforced food sources major for specific individuals. Verdant green vegetables, whole grains, meat, and dairy things are great wellsprings of B supplements.

Magnesium: A Multifunctional Mineral

Magnesium is related with more than 300 biochemical reactions in the body, including muscle and nerve capacity, glucose control, and circulatory strain rule. Nuts, seeds, whole grains, and verdant green vegetables are rich in magnesium, which can help with meeting the extended necessities of those a bigger number of than fifty.

Potassium: Coordinating Circulatory strain

Potassium is basic for staying aware of strong circulatory strain levels, a concern for by far most in their fifties to say the very least. Natural items, vegetables, and vegetables, similar to bananas, sweet potatoes, and beans, are incredible potassium sources, supporting heart prosperity and hindering hypertension.

Water: The Encapsulation of Life

Hydration is fundamental at whatever stage throughout everyday life, but especially for more prepared adults, who could have a decreased sensation of thirst. Water maintains every cell and capacity in the body, including absorption, maintenance of enhancements, and removal of waste. Ensuring good fluid affirmation is essential for by and large prosperity and thriving.

Accommodating Your Eating routine to Your Prerequisites

Understanding these basic enhancements and their importance is the main push toward accommodating your eating routine to meet your healthy necessities after fifty. Uniting an alternate extent of food assortments rich in these enhancements can help with keeping an eye on the extraordinary prosperity challenges and physiological changes of developing, supporting a fiery, sound life.

This part has given a principal perception of the basic enhancements expected for those a larger number of than fifty. Executing this data through dietary choices can fundamentally influence prosperity, centrality, and individual fulfillment in the years to come.

Chapter 3: Reading and Understanding Food Labels: Interpreting Nutritional Information for Smarter Food Choices

In the current market, where food things go with a lot of cases and dietary information, understanding food names is a higher need than any time in ongoing memory. This capacity is particularly key for those a greater number of than fifty, as seeking after informed food choices is pressing for managing prosperity, supporting vitality, and having a tendency to develop unequivocal concerns like heart prosperity, bone thickness, and mental ability. This segment will guide you through the maze of dietary names, helping you with seeking after choices that line up with your prosperity targets.

The Basics of Food Imprints

Food marks give a wealth of information about what's in your food, including its enhancement content, trimmings, and anything is possible from that point. At the focal point of the food mark is the Sustenance Real factors board, which records the serving size, calories, and enhancements like fat, cholesterol, sodium, starches, fiber, sugars, protein, and certain supplements and minerals.

Understanding these parts is the most crucial stage in going with better food choices. For instance, understanding the serving size can help you with estimating the sum you're truly consuming, which is particularly critical for managing calorie utilization and keeping a sound weight.

Key Enhancements to Watch

For those more than fifty, certain enhancements merit excellent thought:

•Fiber: Essential for stomach related prosperity and associated with cut down cholesterol levels, fiber is an enhancement various adults don't get enough of. Look for food sources with high fiber content, similar to whole grains, regular items, and vegetables.

•Sodium: High sodium confirmation can provoke hypertension, a bet factor for coronary sickness. The American Heart Connection recommends something like 2,300 milligrams each day, pushing toward an ideal limitation of something like 1,500 mg every day for most adults.

•Sugars: Added sugars add to a huge gathering of clinical issues, including power and coronary sickness. The Dietary Principles for Americans propose confining calories from added sugars to under 10% of hard and fast calories every day.

•Fats: It is critical to Grasp the sort of fat. Trans fats and inundated fats can raise your bet of coronary disease, while monounsaturated and polyunsaturated fats can maintain heart prosperity.

•Calcium and Vitamin D: Crucial for bone prosperity, these

enhancements are fundamental as you age. Ensure your eating routine consolidates enough of these, especially if you're in peril for osteoporosis.

Unwinding Fixing Records

The trimmings list is also critical as the Food Real factors board. Trimmings are kept in jumping demand by weight, and that suggests the underlying relatively few trimmings make up the weight of the thing. This can help you with avoiding food sources with unwanted added substances or high in sugars and fats. Whole food assortments should ideally be the vital trimmings, rather than sugars or refined grains.

Prosperity Cases and Stamping Terms

Food packaging oftentimes consolidates prosperity cases or checking terms planned to catch your eye, like "low-fat," "high in fiber," or "diminishes cholesterol." Understanding what these terms legitimately mean can help you with making extra taught decisions. For example, "light" or "light" means the thing has 33% less calories or a piece of the fat of the reference food. "Diminished" shows the thing has something like 25% less significantly an enhancement or calories than the reference food.

Helpful Ways of using Food Imprints

1. Start with the Serving Size: Break down the serving size on the imprint to the aggregate you truly eat. Change how you could decipher the fortifying substance considering your serving size.

2. Check the Calories: View at how as a particular food fits into your regular calorie needs, especially if weight the leaders is a goal.

3. Limit Certain Enhancements: Plan to confine doused fats, trans fats, cholesterol, and sodium, which can add to coronary disease and other clinical issues.

4. Seek Out Productive Enhancements: Focus on food sources abundant in dietary fiber, vitamin D, calcium, iron, and potassium, which can maintain prosperity and hinder ailment.
5. Use the Percent Everyday Qualities (%DV): These can help you with understanding how a particular food fits into your everyday eating routine, considering a 2,000 calorie every day diet.

Understanding food marks is a necessary resource for managing your prosperity and sustenance, especially after fifty. By becoming fit in unraveling the information gave on food packaging, you can go with choices that help your dietary necessities, adding to a superior, more unique life. This part has outfitted you with the data to investigate the perplexing universe of food marks, drawing in you to seek after more shrewd food choices that line up with your prosperity targets.

4

Chapter 4: The Balanced Plate: Portions, Food Groups, and How to Create Balanced Meals

Making changed feasts is a workmanship and science that ends up being continuously critical as we age. Our sustaining necessities change, and staying aware of prosperity and significance requires a careful harmony of enhancements from a collection of sustenance types. This part will examine how to divide nourishment types on your plate, promising you get the significant enhancements to help a sound body and mind.

Understanding the Nourishment classes

A sensible eating routine incorporates all the essential nourishment classes: normal items, vegetables, proteins, grains, and dairy (or their different choices). Each get-together offers unique enhancements earnest for prosperity, similar to dietary fiber, key supplements, minerals, and cell fortifications.

•Food varieties developed starting from the earliest stage: for the gold collection, as different assortments address different supplements and cell fortifications. Around half of your plate should be food sources developed starting from the earliest stage each blowout, underlining vegetables over normal items due to their lower sugar content.

•Proteins: Consolidate a combination of protein sources, similar to incline meats, poultry, fish, beans, peas, and nuts. Protein is central for staying aware of mass, which is fundamental as we age.

•Grains: Select whole grains over refined grains, as they give more fiber, which helps with retention and can prevent steady contaminations. Whole grains integrate whole wheat, natural hued rice, oats, and quinoa.

•Dairy or Decisions: Calcium-rich food assortments are basic for bone prosperity. Integrate low-fat or sans fat dairy things, or search for plant-based decisions like almond or soy milk that are stimulated with calcium and vitamin D.

The Possibility of the Sensible Plate

The idea behind the sensible plate is to help with imagining the part sizes and degree of each and every healthful classification you should go all in great gala. Here is an essential strategy for building a sensible plate:

•A part of the plate stacked up with verdant food varieties

•One fourth of the plate with lean protein

•One fourth of the plate with whole grains

•A serving of dairy or a calcium-rich choice as a reconsideration

This approach ensures you're getting a good mix of huge scope and micronutrients in each banquet, supporting as a rule and supervising weight by propelling consummation and diminishing the motivation to glut.

Section Control

Understanding piece sizes is critical for keeping a sound weight and ensuring you're getting an impeccably estimated extent of food. The following are a couple of sensible tips:

•Food sources developed from the beginning: cup of unrefined verdant vegetables or 1/2 cup of cut vegetables or normal item is seen as a serving.

•Proteins: A serving of meat or fish is about the size of a deck of cards or the focal point of your hand.

•Grains: One serving is 1/2 cup of cooked rice, pasta, or oat.

•Dairy: A serving is 1 cup of milk or yogurt or 1.5 ounces of cheddar.

Making Changed Dining experiences

•Breakfast: Start your day with grain polished off with new berries and a side of low-fat yogurt. This banquet gives whole grains, normal item, and dairy, offering a mix of fiber, supplements, and calcium.

•Lunch: A serving of leafy greens with mixed greens, vegetables, chickpeas, a sprinkle of cheddar, and a whole grain roll as an idea in retrospect makes an enhancement thick lunch. You're getting vegetables, protein, dairy, and whole grains in all cases feast.

•Dinner: Grilled salmon with a side of quinoa and steamed broccoli covers your protein, whole grains, and vegetables. Add a glass of supported almond milk to ensure you're getting your calcium.

Adjusting to Express Dietary Necessities

While the fair plate is an unprecedented early phase, it's indispensable to adjust to individual healthy necessities, especially for those with express prosperity concerns like diabetes or coronary disease. For example, someone with diabetes could focus in on lower-carb decisions, while someone stressed over heart prosperity could pick fats adroitly, focusing in on wellsprings of monounsaturated and polyunsaturated fats.

The fair plate model is an astonishing resource for orchestrating feasts that are nutritious, satisfying, and fitting for your dietary necessities as you age. By focusing in on fragment sizes and a mix of nourishing classes, you can ensure that your body is getting the key enhancements it prerequisites to prosper. This part has given the data and realistic direction expected to apply the respectable plate thought to your banquets, supporting a sound, vigorous lifestyle after fifty.

5

Chapter 5: Supplementation: When and How to Use Supplements Effectively and Safely

As we age, our bodies could require extra sustaining help past what our eating routine gives. This can be a result of different components, recollecting changes for handling and supplement maintenance, extended stimulating necessities, or dietary constraints. While food should continually be the important wellspring of enhancements, upgrades can expect a key part in filling feeding openings. In any case, it's pivotal for approach supplementation with care to promise it's done effectively and safely.

Sorting out the Gig of Upgrades

Supplements consolidate supplements, minerals, flavors, amino acids, and proteins gave in various designs like pills, powders, and liquids. Their principal job isn't to replace a sound eating routine anyway to enhance it, ensuring that individuals meet their everyday feeding necessities.

Right when Supplementation May Be Fundamental

•Extended Healthy Necessities: Certain enhancements, similar to vitamin D, calcium, and vitamin B12, become more testing to hold or may be normal in additional critical aggregates as we age.

•Dietary Constraints: Individuals following unequivocal eating regimens (e.g., veggie lover, without gluten) may find it attempting to procure all of the indispensable enhancements from food alone.

•Infirmities: Sicknesses or medications can impact supplement ingestion, making supplements essential to thwart insufficiencies.

Picking the Right Upgrades

•Counsel a Clinical consideration Capable: Preceding starting any improvement, it's crucial to chat with a subject matter expert or an enlisted dietitian. They can propose supplements considering your prosperity status, dietary confirmation, and healthy necessities.

•Quality Matters: Quest for supplements that have been pariah pursued for quality and ideals. Affirmations from affiliations like USP (US Pharmacopeia) or NSF Worldwide show that the thing fulfills serious rules.

•Scrutinize Checks Mindfully: Pick supplements that contain the enhancements you truly need without pointless added substances or fillers. Center around the portion to do whatever it takes not to outperform the recommended ordinary characteristics.

Tips for Secured and Convincing Supplementation

•Follow Proposed Portions: Taking past what the recommended proportion of an upgrade can incite unpleasant effects. Certain supplements and minerals can be hurtful at evident levels.

•Have some familiarity with Correspondences: Upgrades can

help out drugs, affecting their practicality or inciting delayed consequences. Analyze any possible coordinated efforts with your clinical consideration provider.

•Screen Your Improvements: Keep an overview of the general huge number of upgrades you take, including their names, estimations, and the legitimization behind taking them. Share this overview with your clinical consideration provider.

•Screen Your Response: Spotlight on how your body answers an improvement. In case you experience any troublesome effects, quit taking the upgrade and direction your clinical benefits provider.

Central Improvements for Individuals More than Fifty

•Vitamin D and Calcium: Central for bone prosperity, especially as bone thickness lessens with age. Supplementation may be fundamental for those with confined sun transparency and dietary confirmation.

•Vitamin B12: Huge for nerve capacity and the improvement of DNA and red platelets. Supplementation may be required in light of reduced ingestion with age.

•Omega-3 Unsaturated fats: Accommodating for heart prosperity. Supplements like fish oil can be a good decision for individuals who don't consume adequate oily fish.

Upgrades can be a significant gadget for ensuring healthy adequacy, particularly for those more than fifty going up against excellent dietary challenges. Nevertheless, the best approach to convincing and safe supplementation is informed choice and meeting with clinical consideration specialists. By understanding when improvements are significant, picking quality things, and using them cautiously, individuals can maintain their prosperity and success without compromising security.

This part has given a broad framework of how to investigate the confounding universe of upgrades, offering practical direction for coordinating them into your healthy routine proficiently.

6

෧৯ৎ

Chapter 6: The Mediterranean Diet: Benefits, Key Components, and How to Adopt This Lifestyle

The Mediterranean Eating routine is something past a dietary model; it's a lifestyle embraced by people living along the Mediterranean Sea, who have presumably the longest fates on earth. This diet is complimented for its different clinical benefits, particularly for heart prosperity, weight the board, and reducing the bet of steady diseases. Its complement on whole food sources, sound fats, and new trimmings changes immaculately with the refreshing necessities of individuals more than fifty.

Benefits of the Mediterranean Eating schedule

23

Research has dependably exhibited the way that the Mediterranean Eating routine can offer tremendous clinical benefits:

•Heart Prosperity: Lessens the bet of coronary ailment by cutting down circulatory strain and cholesterol levels.

•Weight The board: Supports a sound burden through an eating routine high in fiber and strong fats, which advance satiety.

•Reduced Peril of Consistent Contaminations: Associated with a lower opportunity of type 2 diabetes, Alzheimer's infection, and explicit kinds of illness.

•Further created Life expectancy: Related with a more long future and a predominant individual fulfillment.

Key Pieces of the Mediterranean Eating routine

The Mediterranean Eating routine is portrayed by:

•Results of the dirt: The preparation of every single supper, giving major supplements, minerals, and cell fortifications.

•Whole Grains: Consumed in their whole design, giving fiber and huge enhancements.

•Strong Fats: On a very basic level from olive oil, nuts, and seeds, adding to heart prosperity and for the most part thriving.

•Lean Proteins: Spotlights on fish and poultry over red meat, with fish being a fundamental protein source due to its omega-3 unsaturated fats.

•Vegetables and Nuts: Critical wellsprings of protein, fiber, and sound fats.

•Moderate Dairy: Preferably from matured things like yogurt and cheddar, in moderate aggregates.

•Limited Red Meat and Pastries: Red meat is consumed sparingly, and treats are held for extraordinary occasions.

•Wine With some restriction: Typically one glass every day with feasts, but not required.

Embracing the Mediterranean Lifestyle

Incorporating the Mediterranean Eating routine into your lifestyle incorporates something past changing what you eat; about embracing a perspective spotlights on better norms while never splitting the difference and getting a charge out of banquets as a group, euphoric experience.

1. Start with Vegetables: Mean to fill a piece of your plate with different lovely vegetables at every supper.
2. Switch to Whole Grains: Replace refined grains with whole grains like quinoa, grain, whole wheat, and hearty hued rice.
3. Use Sound Fats: Cook with olive oil as opposed to margarine and goody on nuts instead of taken care of snack food sources.
4. Eat More Fish: Coordinate fish into your suppers something like twice consistently, focusing in on oily fish like salmon, mackerel, and sardines.
5. Enjoy Suppers with Others: Offer banquets with friends and family while possible, making gobbling a social and relaxing experience.
6. Stay Dynamic: Genuine work is a basic piece of the Mediterranean lifestyle. Go all in that you appreciate, such as walking, swimming, or cycling.

Utilitarian Ways of executing the Mediterranean Eating schedule

•Feast Orchestrating: Plan your suppers around vegetables, grains, and lean proteins, including strong fats and dairy with some limitation.

•Shopping Tips: Focus on new, whole food sources, and stock up on staples like olive oil, whole grains, and canned fish for solace.

•Cooking Methodologies: Embrace fundamental cooking strategies like grilling, baking, and sautéing to protect the typical flavors and enhancements of food assortments.

•Cautious Eating: Eat continuously and relish each snack, zeroing in on the flavors and surfaces of your food.

The Mediterranean Eating routine offers a showed method for facilitating created prosperity and success, particularly fit to the sustaining necessities and prosperity stresses of those a larger number of than fifty. By focusing in on whole food sources, sound fats, and lean proteins, and by solidifying the pleasures of shared dining experiences and dynamic work, you can embrace a lifestyle that propels life range, vitality, and delight.

7

Chapter 7: Plant-Based Eating: How to Thrive on a Plant-Based Diet

Embracing a plant-based diet offers an enormous number of clinical benefits, including decreased risks of coronary sickness, hypertension, type 2 diabetes, and certain infections. It moreover lines up with viable eating practices that benefit the planet. This part will guide you through the essentials of plant-based eating, focusing in on promising you help all major enhancements through an especially organized diet and giving model supper plans to inspiration.

The Essentials of Plant-Based Eating

A plant-based diet spins around food sources got from plants, including vegetables, natural items, grains, vegetables, nuts, and seeds, with immaterial or no animal things. The best approach to prospering with this diet is variety, which ensures an enormous number of crucial enhancements.

Key Enhancements and Their Sources

While advancing to a plant-based diet, truly center around the going with supplements:

•Protein: Basic for muscle upkeep and as a rule. Rich plant sources integrate lentils, beans, chickpeas, tofu, tempeh, and quinoa.

•Omega-3 Unsaturated fats: Critical for heart and psyche prosperity. Flaxseeds, chia seeds, walnuts, and hemp seeds are brilliant sources.

•Calcium: Pivotal for bone prosperity. Desire to supported plant milks, tahini, almonds, and green verdant vegetables like kale and broccoli.

•Vitamin B12: Significant for nerve capacity and blood game plan, and ordinarily found in animal things. Consider propped food assortments or a B12 supplement.

•Iron: Plant-based iron (non-heme iron) is found in lentils, beans, reinforced oats, and faint plate of mixed greens. Eating L-ascorbic corrosive rich food assortments nearby iron-rich food assortments can overhaul ingestion.

•Vitamin D: Key for bone prosperity and safe capacity. Beside sunlight transparency, contemplate stimulated food sources or upgrades.

Test Supper Plans

Coming up next are two model day supper means to help you with envisioning how to change a plant-based diet:

Day 1:

•Breakfast: Momentary oats made with supported plant milk, mixed in with chia seeds, polished off with new berries and a spot of almond margarine.

•Lunch: Quinoa salad with dim beans, avocado, cherry tomatoes, corn, and a lime-cilantro dressing.

•Dinner: Skillet burned tofu with broccoli, ringer peppers, and snap peas, served over natural shaded rice, sprinkled with sesame seeds.

•Snacks: Hummus with carrot sticks; a humble bundle of walnuts.

Day 2:

•Breakfast: Smoothie with animated plant milk, spinach, banana, flaxseeds, and mixed berries.

•Lunch: Lentil soup with whole grain bread and a side plate of leafy greens of mixed greens, cucumber, and cherry tomatoes.

•Dinner: Whole wheat pasta with a rich tomato and vegetable sauce, empowering yeast sprinkled on top for a cheddar like flavor.

•Snacks: Apple cuts with peanut butter; a little serving of stewed chickpeas.

Practical Ways of prospering with a Plant-Based Diet

•Plan Your Meals: Assurance combination and balance by orchestrating your banquets. This associates in thinking about each possibility.

•Grasp Imprints: For dealt with plant-based food sources, examining names is crucial to avoid extravagant added sugars and awful fats.

•Supplement Cautiously: Consider supplements for supplements that are attempting to get, as B12 and Vitamin D, following conversing with a clinical benefits provider.

•Stay Informed: Constantly train yourself about plant-based food to go with informed choices about your eating schedule.

Embracing a plant-based diet in your fifties and past can in a general sense add to your prosperity, life length, and success. By focusing in on supplement thick food assortments and ensuring various sources, you can meet your supporting necessities and participate in the wide display of flavors and benefits that plant-based eating offers. This part gives an essential understanding and down to earth gadgets for really coordinating plant-based eating into your lifestyle, focusing on the meaning of balance, variety, and care in dietary choices.

8

Chapter 8:
Anti-Inflammatory Foods: Foods That Fight Inflammation and Support Overall Health

Irritating is the body's normal reaction to injury or disease, a major piece of the recuperating structure. All things considered, constant aggravation can incite or obliterate different clinical issues, including coronary illness, joint disturbance, Alzheimer's torment, and many kinds of hurtful turn of events. Diet expects an epic part in coordinating unsettling influence levels in the body. This section will acquaint you with calming food sources, sort out their advantages, and proposal seminar on the best method for arranging them into your eating routine to help your flourishing as you with developing.

Understanding Unsettling influence and Its Effect

Reliable irritating can be impacted by several parts, including diet, way of life, and normal openings. A directing eating routine spins around food sources that decline the provocative reaction and help with remaining mindful of ideal flourishing.

Key Alleviating Food sources

Several food varieties are known for their alleviating properties. Counting these in your eating routine can assist with reducing worsening levels and safeguard against persistent afflictions:

•Consequences of the soil: Magnificently disguised food sources created beginning from the earliest stage, to berries, oranges, salad greens, and beets, are high in cell strongholds and polyphenols that have alleviating impacts.

•Entire Grains: Food groupings like oat, generous toned rice, and entire wheat bread contain fiber, which can assist with decreasing exacerbation.

•Solid Fats: Wellsprings of omega-3 unsaturated fats, like salmon, chia seeds, flaxseeds, and pecans, are known for their calming properties. Olive oil, particularly extra-virgin olive oil, is solid areas for another food.

•Nuts and Seeds: Almonds, pecans, and seeds like hemp, flax, and chia are wellsprings of solid fats as well as contain cell fortresses that can assist with doing fighting unsettling influence.

•Endlessly enhances: Turmeric, ginger, garlic, and cinnamon are among the flavors known for their directing impacts.

Dietary Models That Tension Reducing Food sources

•The Mediterranean Eating plan: Wealthy in regular things, vegetables, nuts, entire grains, fish, and sound oils, this diet is an astounding model of easing eating.

•Plant-Based Diets: Featuring food groupings from plant sources regularly prompts an eating routine high in easing compounds.

Planning Calming Food arrangements into Your Eating schedule

Taking on an easing diet shouldn't worry about a total update of your dietary models for the present. Little, reasonable changes for quite a while can have an immense effect:

1. Increase Verdant food sources Affirmation: Hold nothing back five servings of aftereffects of the soil consistently, zeroing in on mix and grouping.
2. Choose Entire Grains Over Refined: Trade out white bread, pasta, and rice for their entire grain accessories.
3. Incorporate Sound Fats: Utilize olive oil for cooking and dressing servings of mixed greens, nibble on nuts, and recall sleek fish for your dinners two times reliably.
4. Spice It Up: Add easing flavors like turmeric and ginger to your occasions for flavor and clinical advantages.
5. Stay Hydrated: Water keeps up with all body limits, including the evacuation of poisons that can add to exacerbation.

Test Feasting experience Contemplations

•Breakfast: Oats finished with pecans, berries, and a sprinkle of cinnamon.

•Lunch: A tremendous serving of salad greens with blended greens, vegetables, chickpeas, avocado, and a dressing made with olive oil and lemon juice.

•Supper: Barbecued salmon with a side of quinoa and steamed broccoli, prepared with garlic and ginger.

•Snacks: Almonds, carrot sticks with hummus, or new typical thing.

Coordinating easing food combinations into your eating routine is a proactive step towards overseeing irritating and supporting your general flourishing. By zeroing in on a tight eating routine well off in typical things, vegetables, entire grains, sound fats, and flavors, you can assist with safeguarding your body against the impacts of consistent unsettling influence and overhaul your prosperity as you age. This portion has equipped you with the information and reasonable tips to embrace calming eating, making it an anticipated and boggling piece of your way of life.

Chapter 9: Food Allergies and Intolerances: Navigating Dietary Restrictions and Alternatives

Food sensitivities and bigotries can fundamentally influence dietary decisions and sustenance. As we age, the body's reaction to specific food sources can change, once in a while bringing about new responsive qualities. This part investigates how to deal with these difficulties really, guaranteeing a reasonable and nutritious eating regimen while keeping away from tricky food sources.

Grasping Food Sensitivities and Prejudices

•Food Sensitivities happen when the safe framework responds to a particular food protein as a danger, causing side effects that can go from gentle to perilous.

•Food Bigotries, like lactose narrow mindedness, don't include the invulnerable framework however can cause inconvenience and stomach related issues.

Recognizing which food sources cause antagonistic responses is pivotal for dealing with these circumstances. Normal allergens incorporate nuts, shellfish, dairy, and wheat.

Procedures for Overseeing Dietary Limitations

1. Identification and Finding: Work with a medical services proficient to distinguish sensitivities and bigotries. This might include keeping a food journal, end diets, and clinical trials.
2. Reading Marks: Become capable in perusing food names to recognize stowed away allergens and risky fixings. Regulation in numerous nations expects allergens to be plainly recorded on bundling.
3. Finding Other options: For each food you should stay away from, there's possible a protected other option. Investigate choices like sans lactose dairy items, without gluten grains, and plant-based protein sources.
4. Meal Preparation and Readiness: Arranging feasts ahead of time and planning food at home can make overseeing sensitivities and prejudices simpler, guaranteeing you have protected and nutritious choices accessible.

Dietary Contemplations

Keeping away from specific food varieties can prompt nourishing holes. For instance, dairy gives calcium and vitamin D, while entire grains are a decent wellspring of B nutrients and fiber. Finding elective hotspots for these supplements is fundamental. Enhancements might be essential however ought to be viewed if all else fails and picked under the direction of a medical care proficient.

Protected and Fulfilling Dietary Other options

•Dairy Sensitivities and Bigotries: Plant-based milks and dairy options, like almond, soy, and oat milk, are sustained with calcium and vitamin D.

•Gluten Awareness and Celiac Illness: sans gluten grains like quinoa, rice, and buckwheat offer incredible options in contrast to wheat, grain, and rye.

•Nut Sensitivities: Seeds, similar to sunflower or pumpkin seeds, can supplant nuts in numerous recipes, giving comparative healthful advantages without the gamble.

•Egg Sensitivities: For baking, consider substitutes like fruit purée, squashed banana, or business egg replacers.

Down to earth Ways to eat Out

Eating out with food sensitivities or bigotries requires alert:

•Convey Your Requirements: Obviously clear up your dietary limitations for eatery staff.

•Pick Astutely: Decide on foundations that are known for obliging dietary limitations.

•Remain Informed: Use applications and online assets that offer data on sensitivity agreeable cafés and food varieties.

Exploring food sensitivities and prejudices requires carefulness and arranging, however it doesn't need to restrict your satisfaction in food. By recognizing dangerous food sources, figuring out how to understand marks, and finding nutritious other options, you can keep a reasonable eating routine that upholds your wellbeing and prosperity. This section has given the instruments and information to oversee dietary limitations successfully, guaranteeing that you can keep on flourishing regardless of these difficulties.

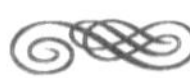

Chapter 10: Eating for Energy: Foods that Boost Energy and How to Incorporate Them into Daily Meals

As we investigate our fifties to say the least, staying aware of high energy levels can end up being logically troublesome. The food sources we eat expect a basic part in our energy levels, influencing how we feel throughout the day. This part plunges into such food assortments that can regularly help energy and offers course on incorporating them into your eating routine to help upheld centrality.

Understanding Energy-Aiding Food assortments

Energy-helping food assortments are those that give a reliable supply of fuel to the body, ideally through a mix of incredible starches, strong fats, and proteins. They also contain supplements and minerals that are major for energy absorption.

•Complex Starches: Food assortments like whole grains, natural items, and vegetables give a steady appearance of glucose into the flow framework, offering upheld energy.

•Sound Fats: Sources like avocados, nuts, seeds, and olive oil add to longer-getting through energy levels without the spikes and plunges related with high-sugar food sources.

•Proteins: Lean proteins from plant and animal sources help in the slow appearance of energy and are central for muscle fix and advancement.

•Hydration: Good water affirmation is huge for ideal energy levels as even delicate parchedness can incite exhaustion.

Food sources to Solidify for Further developed Energy

•Whole Grains: Quinoa, hearty shaded rice, and oats are surprising for upheld energy. They're affluent in fiber, helping with overseeing glucose levels.

•Salad Greens: Spinach, kale, and Swiss chard are high in iron, an imperative part in energy creation, especially huge for women.

•Nuts and Seeds: Almonds, walnuts, and chia seeds are energy-thick, giving strong fats, proteins, and fiber.

•Natural items: Berries, apples, and oranges offer ordinary sugars and fiber for a quick shock of energy without the mishap that comes from took care of sugar.

•Vegetables: Beans and lentils are remarkable protein sources as well as affluent in complex starches and fiber, progressing upheld energy release.

Test Supper Contemplations for Upheld Energy

•Breakfast: Momentary oats with chia seeds, berries, and a spoonful of almond spread for a blend of complex carbs, sound fats, and protein.

•Lunch: A quinoa salad with mixed vegetables, chickpeas, and a lemon-tahini dressing, offering a fair mix of protein, fiber, and sound fats.

•Dinner: Grilled chicken or tofu with a side of hearty shaded rice and steamed broccoli, giving areas of strength for an of protein, complex carbs, and supplements.

•Snacks: Cut apples with peanut butter or an unobtrusive pack of mixed nuts for rapid, nutritious shocks of energy.

Ways of intensifying Energy through Diet

1. Balance Your Banquets: Pull out all the stops of complex carbs, sound fats, and proteins to supply ensure a reliable energy.
2. Stay Hydrated: Hydrate throughout the day to prevent the energy-depleting effects of parchedness.
3. Limit Sweet Food sources: Reduce confirmation of high-sugar things that can provoke energy spikes followed by crashes.
4. Mind Your Pieces: Glutting can provoke lethargy, while too little food can achieve a shortfall of energy. Find the right harmony for your development level.

Embracing an eating routine well off in energy-helping food sources can in a general sense influence your centrality and ability to keep a working lifestyle. By focusing in on whole, supplement thick food sources and ensuring changed meals, you can see the value in upheld energy levels throughout the day. This segment has given the data and mechanical assemblies to help you with incorporating these food assortments into your eating standard, empowering you to thrive with noteworthiness and energy.

11

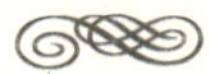

Chapter 11: Hydration: The Role of Water in Health and How to Ensure Adequate Intake

Hydration expects a fundamental part in staying aware of prosperity, influencing everything from cell capacity and skin prosperity to mental execution and stomach related prosperity. As we age, our body's ability to screen water diminishes, and our sensation of thirst could end up being less extreme, making parchedness a more basic bet with potentially serious outcomes. This part includes the meaning of hydration, the clinical benefits of water, and rational ways of ensuring you're sufficiently hydrated.

Sorting out the Meaning of Hydration

Water is principal everlastingly, drew in with numerous actual cycles, including:

•Overseeing inner intensity level

•Transporting enhancements and oxygen

•Taking out waste and toxins

•Lubing up joints

•Supporting stomach related prosperity

Drying out can incite a lot of clinical issues, from minor incidental effects like headaches and exhaustion to extra outrageous conditions, for instance, kidney stones, urinary bundle sicknesses, and, shockingly, prevented mental capacity.

How Much Water Do You Need?

How much water a solitary necessities can move considering factors like age, weight, climate, and development level. While the "8x8" rule (eight 8-ounce glasses of water every day) is a good normal standard, prerequisites can move. It's moreover crucial to observe that all fluids add to hydration, including water, milk, crush, and even coffee and tea. Food varieties developed starting from the earliest stage have high water content and can help add to your overall fluid affirmation.

Ways of staying Hydrated

1. Start Your Day with Water: Begin consistently with a glass of water to send off hydration.

2. Carry a Water Holder: Keeping a water bottle with you can remind you to take standard preferences throughout the span of the day.

3. Eat Water-Rich Food sources: Coordinate results of the dirt like cucumbers, tomatoes, oranges, and watermelons into your eating routine.

4. Set Updates: Use wireless applications or set alerts as ideas to hydrate at typical ranges.

5. Monitor Your Pee: Light to light yellow pee regularly shows

authentic hydration, while faint pee can be a sign of parchedness.

Seeing Signs of Drying out

It's fundamental to see the signs of absence of hydration, which can include:

•Thirst

•Dry mouth

•Exhaustion

•Befuddlement

•Less customary pee

More settled adults, explicitly, should be mindful about staying aware of hydration as they wouldn't really in all cases feel dried regardless, when the body needs fluids.

Keeping an eye on Hydration Hardships

For certain's motivations, drinking agreeable fluids can challenge. Here are methodology to overcome ordinary obstructions:

•If you could manage without the kind of plain water, have a go at adding a cut of lemon, lime, cucumber, or a sprinkle of normal item squeeze for some additional punch.

•If you find it hard to try to hydrate, convey a water compartment or set reports on your phone.

Palatable hydration is a groundwork of good prosperity, especially as we age. By understanding the fundamental work water plays in our regularphysical processes, seeing the signs of drying out, and using frameworks to augment fluid confirmation, we can maintain our overall flourishing and vitality. This segment has given the data and gadgets essential to zero in on hydration in your everyday prosperity schedule, ensuring that you stay by and large around hydrated and thrive.

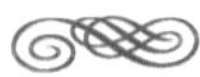

Chapter 12: Meal Planning and Prep: Strategies for Success, Including Sample Meal Plans and Recipes

Sensible feasting experience coordinating and organizing are key to supporting a sound eating schedule, particularly for those in their fifties no doubt. By organizing dinners early, you can guarantee that you're eating a good eating standard, set aside an open door and cash, and reduce food squander. This fragment will walk you through the technique for useful dinner sorting out and prepare, trailed by test feast plans and recipes that line up with the solid essentials and dietary models talked about in past parts.

The Nuts and bolts of Dinner Coordinating

1. Assess Your Supporting Requirements: Ponder your success

objectives, dietary obstructions, and a particular solid necessities considering your age, movement level, and clinical issue.

2. Choose Your Dinner Coordinating Style: Close whether you like to setup eats bit by bit or fortnightly and whether pack cooking or regular arrangement turns out to be brutal for you.

3. Gather Recipes: Gather recipes that fit your dietary necessities and individual taste. Select recipes that have an equilibrium of vegetables, protein, and solid fats.

4. Make a Shopping Outline: taking into account your picked recipes, make a shopping synopsis to guarantee you buy every single crucial fixing.

Frameworks for Dinner Prep Achievement

•Pack Cooking: Plan tremendous parts of express dishes that can be dealt with and eaten dependably, like soups, stews, and goulashes.

•Prep Decorations Early: Wash and hack vegetables, marinate proteins, and part out snacks near the start of the week to save time on elaborate days.

•Utilize the Cooler: Freeze bits of organized feasts for a long time whenever you want the opportunity to cook.

•Put resources into Quality Holders: Having various sizes for limit compartments can make spreading and dealing with feasts not so much intricate but rather more obliging.

Test Dinner Plan

Day 1:

•Breakfast: Spinach and Feta Omelet with Entire Grain Toast

•Lunch: Quinoa Salad with Burned Vegetables and Chickpeas

•Supper: Barbecued Salmon with Steamed Broccoli and Yam

•Snacks: Almonds; Greek Yogurt with Honey and Berries

Day 2:

•Breakfast: Transient Oats with Chia Seeds, Almond Spread, and Banana

•Lunch: Turkey and Avocado Wrap; Blended Green Plate of salad greens in with Olive Oil and Lemon Dressing

•Supper: Chicken Sautéed food with Generous shaded Rice and Blended Vegetables

•Snacks: Cut Cucumber with Hummus; Apple Cuts

Test Recipes

Quinoa Salad with Burned Vegetables and Chickpeas

•Decorations: 1 cup quinoa, 2 cups blended vegetables (e.g., cost peppers, zucchini, cherry tomatoes), 1 can chickpeas (depleted and flushed), olive oil, lemon juice, salt, pepper, feta cheddar (discretionary).

•Rules: Cook quinoa as shown by bunch headings. Cook vegetables in the stove with olive oil, salt, and pepper until delicate. Blend cooked quinoa, stewed vegetables, and chickpeas. Dress with olive oil, lemon press, salt, and pepper. Top with feta cheddar whenever required.

Barbecued Salmon with Steamed Broccoli and Yam

•Decorations: Salmon filets, broccoli florets, 1 yam, olive oil, lemon, flavors (e.g., dill or parsley), salt, pepper.

•Rules: Season salmon with olive oil, lemon, flavors, salt, and pepper; barbecue until cooked through. Steam broccoli and force a yam until touchy. Serve salmon with a side of broccoli and yam.

Dinner coordinating and status are connected to some unique choice from picking what to eat; they're associated with pursuing purposeful decisions that help your thriving and way of life targets. This part gives an establishment to arranging incredible thinning down inclinations into your normal everyday arrangement, with approaches and recipes expected to improve the association and confirmation you're supporting your body with the right food varieties. By carving out an opportunity to endlessly design, you can see the worth in tasty, nutritious dinners that fuel your body and work on your prosperity.

13

Chapter 13: Staying on Track: Tips for Dining Out, Travel, and Maintaining Nutrition Goals Amid a Busy Lifestyle

Keeping a nutritious eating routine while feasting out, voyaging, or dealing with a chaotic timetable can appear to be overwhelming. Notwithstanding, with the right techniques, you can partake in these encounters without crashing your wellbeing and sustenance objectives. This part gives tips to pursuing informed food decisions in different circumstances, guaranteeing that you can remain focused regardless of where life takes you.

Feasting Out

•See the Menu: Take a gander at the menu online early on to settle on a solid choice without the strain of requesting on the spot.

•Request Changes: Feel free to for dishes to be ready in a better manner, for example, barbecuing as opposed to broiling or dressing as an afterthought.

•Watch Part Sizes: Eatery bits can be liberal. Think about sharing a dish or requesting half to be taken care of ahead of time.

Voyaging

•Pack Bites: Bring sound tidbits like nuts, natural products, and entire grain saltines to try not to depend on air terminal or side of the road choices.

•Remain Hydrated: Convey a water jug to guarantee you stay hydrated, particularly during air travel.

•Research Neighborhood Cooking: Distinguish solid choices commonplace of your objective that will permit you to appreciate nearby flavors without compromising nourishment.

Occupied Way of life

•Dinner Prep: Devote time every week to plan feasts ahead of time. Having solid choices promptly accessible can forestall last-minute unfortunate decisions.

•Solid Eating: Keep sound snacks at your work environment or in your sack to control hunger and try not to distribute machine enticements.

•Adaptable Dinner Arranging: Have an adaptable feast plan that can adjust to surprising changes in your timetable.

Adjusting Delight and Wellbeing

•Practice Careful Eating: Spotlight on the experience of eating. Relish the flavors and surfaces, and pay attention to your body's yearning and completion signs.

•Balance Is Vital: It's OK to periodically enjoy. What makes the biggest difference is the general example of your eating routine.

•Excuse Yourself: On the off chance that you stray from your sustenance objectives, don't be too unforgiving with yourself. Recognize it, gain from the experience, and refocus with your next feast.

Remaining Roused

•Put forth Practical Objectives: Put forth reachable sustenance objectives that empower progress without setting you up for disappointment.

•Keep tabs on Your Development: Keeping a food journal or utilizing a sustenance application can assist you with remaining mindful of your dietary patterns and progress towards your objectives.

•Look for Help: Offer your nourishment objectives with companions or relatives who can offer help and responsibility.

Exploring feasting out, travel, and a bustling way of life while keeping up with sustenance objectives requires arranging, adaptability, and a fair methodology. By utilizing the methodologies framed in this section, you can partake in the delights of food and different culinary encounters without undermining your wellbeing. Keep in mind, the objective is to pursue decisions that help your prosperity and fit inside the system of a reasonable eating regimen, permitting you to flourish at whatever stage in life.

Conclusion: Empowerment Through Nutrition: Encouragement and Final Thoughts on Living a Vibrant, Healthy Life After 50

The excursion through "Fifty and Flourishing" has been one of disclosure, understanding, and arrangement. As you stand at this point, outfitted with an abundance of information on nourishment, hydration, feast arranging, and the significance of a reasonable eating routine, you are more than prepared to embrace a way of life that broadens your years as well as enhances them with quality and delight.

The Force of Decision

Consistently, we go with decisions about what to eat, how to invest our energy, and which propensities to develop. These decisions shape our wellbeing, impact our prosperity, and decide the course of our lives as we age. Picking healthfully rich food sources, remaining hydrated, and participating in ordinary actual work are demonstrations of sense of pride and taking care of oneself that significantly affect our imperativeness and wellbeing.

Sustenance as a Mainstay of Wellbeing

Sustenance is something other than fuel for our bodies; it's an establishment for a dynamic life. The food sources we eat can either add to the advancement of illnesses or go about as preventive medication. In your grasp lies the ability to fundamentally impact your wellbeing results. Embrace this power with energy and a pledge to feeding your body with what it genuinely needs.

Living Energetically After 50

Maturing is an unavoidable piece of life, yet the way in which we age is to a great extent inside our control. The account of decline as we age is one that we have the ability to revise. By zeroing in on nourishment and pursuing decisions that help our physical and psychological wellness, we can keep on living energetically, with energy, strength, and lucidity, a ways into our later years.

The Excursion Ahead

As you push ahead, recollect that the excursion to keeping a sound way of life is progressing. There will be difficulties and misfortunes, yet each step you take towards embracing a better eating regimen and way of life is a stage towards a seriously satisfying life. Permit yourself beauty and adaptability. Wellbeing isn't about flawlessness yet about settling on additional empowering decisions more regularly.

A Last Expression of Consolation

You have every one of the devices you want to flourish. With information, assurance, and a feeling of self-sympathy, there is no restriction to what you can accomplish in your wellbeing process. Let "Fifty and Flourishing" be your aide, in sustenance as well as in taking on a point of view that is loaded with plausibility, development, and happiness.

May this guide act as a reference point of light on your way, enlightening the way towards a future where you're getting by as well as flourishing. Embrace the experience of living great, for the greatest long stretches of your life are not behind you — they are occurring at present, ready with potential and ready to be seized with two hands.

Appendices

Glossary of Terms

- **Antioxidants**: Compounds found in food that can prevent or slow damage to cells caused by free radicals, thereby reducing inflammation and the risk of chronic diseases.
- **Complex Carbohydrates**: Carbohydrates consisting of long chains of sugar molecules; found in foods such as whole grains, vegetables, and legumes. They provide sustained energy and are rich in fiber.
- **Dehydration**: A condition that occurs when the loss of body fluids, mostly water, exceeds the amount taken in. It can lead to decreased energy and impaired bodily functions.
- **Macronutrients**: The main nutrients required by the human body to produce energy, including carbohydrates, proteins, and fats.
- **Micronutrients**: Vitamins and minerals required by the body in small amounts for proper functioning and disease prevention.
- **Omega-3 Fatty Acids**: A type of essential fatty acid known for supporting heart health, cognitive function, and reducing inflammation.
- **Probiotics**: Live bacteria and yeasts beneficial to the digestive system, often referred to as "good" bacteria.
- **Sarcopenia**: The loss of skeletal muscle mass and strength as a result of aging.

- **Whole Foods**: Foods that are processed and refined as little as possible, presented in their natural form.

Resources for Further Reading

- **Books**:
    - "How Not to Die" by Michael Greger, M.D.: An exploration of how nutritional choices impact our health and longevity.
    - "Eat, Drink, and Be Healthy" by Walter Willett, M.D.: Provides insights into the Harvard Healthy Eating Pyramid and offers practical advice on healthy eating.
    - "The Blue Zones Solution" by Dan Buettner: Investigates communities worldwide where people live the longest and offers lessons for living a long and healthy life.
- **Websites**:
    - Harvard School of Public Health – Nutrition Source: Offers a wealth of information on nutrition, healthy eating, and guidelines for disease prevention.
    - EatRight.org (Academy of Nutrition and Dietetics): Provides resources on nutrition and health, including tips for aging adults.
    - MedlinePlus – Nutrition: A resource for reliable, up-to-date health information on nutrition from the National Institutes of Health.
- **Organizations**:
    - **Academy of Nutrition and Dietetics**: The world's largest organization of food and nutrition professionals, offering education and advocacy.
    - **American Heart Association**: Provides guidelines and information on heart-healthy eating patterns.

These resources are intended to supplement the information provided in "Fifty & Thriving" and encourage further exploration into the topics of nutrition, health, and wellness. Whether you're seeking to deepen your understanding of specific dietary patterns, looking for healthy recipes, or wanting to stay updated on the latest nutrition research, these resources can provide valuable support.